Anti-Inflammatory
Elimination Diet
Health Food Plan

(The O Diet)

Your Guide to 3 Allergy-Free Steps For
Discovering Food Allergies and
Developing a Healthy Anti-Inflammatory
Diet For Life

~

Veronica Bond, RDN, LDN

Eye on Life Publications

Anti-Inflammatory Elimination Diet Health Food Plan
Copyright © 2015 Veronica Bond

ISBN 10: 150023107X
ISBN 13: 978-1500231071

Disclaimer: The information contained within this book is not intended to be a substitute for professional clinical advice. Only a qualified professional can undertake diagnosis and treatment of any clinical condition. Readers of this book should always seek the advice of a qualified health professional with any questions they have regarding their health or a medical condition. Neither the author nor the publisher guarantees the accuracy, quality, suitability or reliability of any information contained in this book.

Other Books by Veronica Bond

Healing Your Inner Child and Yourself For Life:
Your Guide to Happiness, Healing Your Heart's
Wounds and Loving Yourself When You Don't Know
How

Money Manifesting Power:
The 5 Most Powerful Ways You Block Your Wealth
How to Overcome Them and Start Attracting Money
For Life

Table of Contents

Table of Contents

Introduction

~**

I want to thank you for taking the first step to better health by picking up this handy guide! In it you will learn step-by-step, exactly how to diagnose any allergic or inflammatory reactions you may be having to certain "every day" foods we typically don't think twice about eating regularly. You may even be taking over-the-counter or prescription drugs on a regular basis to relieve your symptoms.

I've created this informative booklet to guide people who are suffering through the three easy steps of the Oligoantigenic Anti-Inflammatory Diet plan, complete with suggested meal plans for great success. With this plan, identifying the trigger foods that cause *your* allergenic symptoms has never been easier!

What is the Oligoantigenic Diet?

The Oligoantigenic Diet (The O Diet) is an inexpensive 3-step process of elimination meal plan, where you closely monitor the effects the foods you're eating have on your body. Originally developed and used in the United Kingdom for identifying food allergies in children, this diagnostic meal plan has proven in recent years to be quite beneficial in helping adults all over the world as well. The diet is prescribed in a range of modifications, but the version that's most effective for *accurately* identifying food allergies is highly recommended.

When your immune system thinks the ingredient(s) of a particular food is a potential threat to your health, it causes your body to react, and you become aware of this through certain symptoms. If you suffer consistently from conditions like a running nose, asthma or breathing problems, migraines, sinus issues, arthritis, skin irritation, eczema, irritable bowel syndrome, attention-deficit disorder (ADHD), depression, mood swings, etc., it's more than likely that you could be allergic to one or more of the "every day" foods you may eat or drink on a regular basis.

Due to variations in frequency and moderation, it can sometimes be difficult to recognize which foods may be causing these symptoms; this is why many of us go undiagnosed for years, seeing doctors, popping pills, battling allergies that could disappear overnight if we only knew we were allergic to eggs, or chicken, or milk, or any number of other common foods.

So this handy step-by-step booklet will be a guide to help you with the process of effectively diagnosing whether or not you're allergic to specific foods.

Now, I know that 'Oligoantigenic' is a mouthful! But to break it down simply, the diet has this name because 'oligo' basically means few, and 'antigenic' is a substance that triggers the production of an antibody.

Note: The O Diet is NOT a starvation or weight loss program.

Is the O Diet Safe?

Yes. An increasing number of positive results from clinical studies show the 3-step O Diet works like a cure for diagnosing food allergies. Health regulators and relevant research organizations have made concessions on the fact that the O Diet, if followed, can stabilize gastrointestinal inflammation. Since cases of food allergies are on the rise in the United States, regulatory authorities are still researching the diet's effectiveness through ongoing and controlled studies.

According to Dr. Paolo Lionetti of the department of pediatrics at Meyer Children Hospital at the University of Florence, allergies could be on the rise due to a *decrease* in the number of gut bacteria in Western people.

Why We're Allergic to Some Foods but Not Others

With what we know about allergenic foods to date, it's helpful to thoroughly understand the basics about food allergies as you prepare to start the O Diet plan.

As we've said, food hypersensitivity inflames your gut, and can cause a myriad of annoying symptoms, including mild to severe migraines, irritable bowel syndrome (IBS), chronic anal fissures, gastrointestinal disorders, Crohn's disease, and many other problems.

Believe it or not, the very center of our immune system is in our gut! A very large percentage of our body's immune activity occurs in the digestive system. Your immune system is always on high alert, so as soon as you put any food into your mouth, your body's defense mechanisms begin evaluating the ingredients in order to safeguard your wellbeing.

But sometimes your immune system takes a food as a harmful substance by mistake, and immediately releases antibodies, known as immunoglobulin E, to neutralize the perceived negative effects the food may have on your body. So, whenever you eat even a slight amount of that particular ingredient, the immunoglobulin E informs your immune system to release a chemical called histamine into the bloodstream.

The release of histamine and other similar chemicals in your blood *causes the allergic symptoms*. That's when you get the itchy eyes, sinus pressure, the skin rashes, dry throat, nausea, asthma, migraines, ____ (insert symptoms that plague you!)

And with that foundation laid, let's get started. Please proceed to Step #1 of the O Diet!

Step #1: Cleaning House – The Forbidden Foods

~

Step 1 is all about being vigilant and removing specific "high risk" foods from your daily diet. You'll begin by ignoring the food items that are most associated with potentially causing an allergic response in the body. Now, you might feel a little uncomfortable at this stage because most of the foods or food ingredients that you're crazy about are going to disappear from your diet. But the plus side is, it's only for two weeks. So relax.

This process will give your digestive system a much-needed break so it can relax and reset itself. A minimum of two weeks is needed to allow your body to adjust and be cleansed of any current irritants. The food elements your body is habitually digesting will no longer be present, allowing any inflammation in your gut to subside and reduce discomfort.

This shift in your diet pattern is quite safe, as you are simply eliminating the foods that can possibly cause an abnormal immune response. And remember, it's only for two weeks, unless you wish to make it three or more. So you can do it!

The types of food to <u>AVOID</u> on the O Diet are those that are most commonly known to be associated with digestion irritation or inflammation. Don't be intimidated. Your quality of life is well worth it!

* NO foods containing artificial colors or flavors - these are powerful triggers

* NO cheese

* NO chocolates or candies

* NO fish

* NO chicken

* NO veal

* NO pork

* NO wheat, oat, barley, corn or cereal

* NO corn, nut, vegetable or soya oils

* NO dairy products at all - no cow's milk, goat milk, butter, margarine, eggs, yogurt, etc.

* NO fruits

* NO sugar, honey, yeast products, spices, or preservatives

* NO nuts, peanuts, almonds, cashews, etc.

* NO peanut butter, jellies, cream cheese, etc.

Drinks to Avoid:

* NO tea, coffee, orange juice or other citrus drinks, apple juice, grape juice, carbonated drinks or sodas, mixed drinks, etc.

* NO alcohol, especially red wine or beer

Some of the forbidden items may surprise you! Most people tend to think that chicken is always a healthy option, but that's not true in this case. Studies have shown that some people are very much allergic to poultry products. Chicken is known to cause allergy symptoms like nasal congestion, fever, ear infection, migraine, watery eyes, nausea, cramps and hives. Chicken can even cause breathing complications.

Some processed meats like hot dogs, nuggets, corned beef, and meats found in canned soups, etc., are typically made of hydrolyzed wheat protein or non-fat dry milk. These are all allergenic ingredients.

So, remember, for Step #1 of the O Diet, you'll be eliminating all of the above food items.

The Easiest Ways to Avoid the Allergenic or Trigger Foods

Our taste buds know what they like, and that's why changing our eating habits all at once tends to be very difficult. So here are some VERY helpful tips for avoiding the forbidden foods, and for developing a taste for the hypoallergenic replacements coming up in Step #2 of the O Diet. You can actually make some very good, mouthwatering recipes out of them!

• Read labels carefully for forbidden ingredients when grocery shopping

• Try to eat in the same place every day

• If a spouse, kids or other family members are eating the forbidden foods, prepare your hypoallergenic meal FIRST and wash your utensils thoroughly; also, try not to eat when they do, to avoid temptation (but remember, it's temporary!)

• Avoid pantry mix up. Label your food ingredients as "safe" and "not safe" for your convenience

• Your house should be free of any allergenic food residues. Tell your family members to wash their hands thoroughly after every meal

• Change your garbage bag daily

• It's best to avoid eating out during the O Diet, but if you *must,* try to call the restaurant and ask about any non-allergenic menu items; stick to basics and be sure to double check about the ingredients before you decide what to order

• When traveling, be sure to inform your airline or hotel staff about your dietary needs in advance

Note: Any initial discomfort and cravings during Step #1 of the O Diet should subside in the first week as your body stabilizes. And fear not. You will be re-introducing all of these forbidden foods to your diet, one at a time in Step #3.

But for now, let's proceed to Step #2!

Step #2: Your New Menu – Hypoallergenic Foods ONLY For Two Weeks

~

Now we're ready for Step #2. After learning which foods you'll be putting on pause for two consecutive weeks, the second step is entirely focused on what you CAN eat! These are foods that contain healthy nutrients and are typically safe for adults of any age and children as well.

You will get to eat *some* fruits, green vegetables and proteins!

You will be eating what's known as hypoallergenic foods. These are foods that have been scientifically proven to contain the *least* amount of inflammatory substances, and pose little to no threat to our digestion and immune system. They are not generally known to cause bloating, swelling, constipation, or any other such related dietary symptoms. Do keep in mind, though, that there are some exceptions. A small percentage of people can even be allergic to these foods.

Note: There is NO exception to this diet plan. The forbidden trigger foods are out, and the safe foods are in. You should also take a multivitamin supplement if you don't already.

The Foods You <u>CAN</u> Eat on the Oligoantigenic Diet

First, the Cruciferous Vegetables:

• Broccoli, cabbage, cauliflower, collard greens, Brussels sprouts, kale, turnips, kohlrabi and rutabaga. These vegetables are considered safest to start with.

• You can also have carrots, parsnips, and lettuce

Next, the Meat Options:

• Lamb (best for your digestive system!)
• Beef

How About Starches? You may be surprised to learn that you're allowed to have:

• Potatoes

• White rice

Cooking Oils:

• Extra virgin olive oil

• Sunflower oil

Fruit Options:

• Bananas

• Apples

• Pears

What You Can Drink:

• Water (that's it!)

Are you wondering if you can stick to this list for two whole weeks? Well, you can't actually find out what in your regular diet could be causing allergy symptoms until you take this step. And guess what, your digestive system will welcome the break as well!

Note: There can be some exceptions per individual on the allowed food list. If you have severe bowel issues, you may want to avoid the cabbage and Brussels sprouts.

Grab your calendar and pick a date to begin your O Diet. I recommend starting on a Monday, the beginning of a fresh workweek, even if you're retired or do not work at all.

Next up, I have some menu ideas that you can follow for good results. However, these are not compulsory schedules. You can always alter the arrangement of the <u>allowed</u> foods to suit your own tastes. And you may use salt and pepper for seasoning.

Note: Due to the limited number of allowed foods, it's best to adjust to eating any of the food choices at any time of the day, verses the traditional eating habits like "breakfast foods" in the mornings.

Suggested Meal Plans
For the O Diet

Hypoallergenic Menu Plan - Day 1

Breakfast: Have some rice and broccoli with a sliced pear

Lunch: Cut up a hamburger patty in a nice green salad with a drizzle of extra virgin olive oil

Dinner: You can try lamb stew with potatoes and carrots, and a green salad on the side. Don't forget to make all salads using the recommended vegetables only

Hypoallergenic Menu Plan - Day 2

Breakfast: Make a nice banana smoothie using ice and water

Lunch: Green salad, carrot sticks, and a sliced apple

Dinner: Pot roast and potatoes; season to taste, but minimally

Hypoallergenic Menu Plan - Day 3

Breakfast: Chopped beef sausages and mashed potatoes

Lunch: Paleo Flax Tortillas with a tasty shredded lamb filling. (Paleo Flax Tortillas are free of grain, egg, corn, gluten, nuts and soy. You can moisten them with olive or sunflower oil)

Dinner: You can have a pepper steak green salad with sliced apples

Rinse and repeat. You can map out the next eleven days with your own variations as you find what works best for your tastes, schedule, etc.

Snack options will be limited to more bananas, apples or pears. You may also have quick helpings of beef or lamb soup! Also cabbage, potato, carrot, or rice soup.

Note: I know this is probably the last thing you want to hear, but in some extreme cases, there are those who are allergic even to apples, pears or bananas. So if you like, you can take a more radical form of the O Diet by having only one (or none) of these fruits for the full two weeks, and then including the others in Step #3.

Remember, it's only temporary and all for your good! Hang in there - you *can* do it!

* ~*

Now, grab a journal and head on into Step #3, the final phase of the O Diet journey!

Step #3: Finding the Culprit – Reintroducing the Forbidden Foods One-by-One

~

Now it's time to systematically bring back those pesky trigger foods, which are probably the ones you were used to eating the most. But mind you, you will not be eating them all at once.

You'll need a journal. Or you can even use a calendar. You will be eating one trigger food item <u>every three days</u> after two full weeks on the O Diet. You will need to write down the food item you're reintroducing, and it should be the ONLY forbidden food you add back into your diet. This is *very* important to the diagnostic process.

Absolutely NO exceptions.

You will watch yourself closely for any mild to severe allergic reactions in your body. Is the immune response fast, or is it slow? You're basically monitoring yourself and allowing your body to tell you what foods it's allergic to.

A person with a hyperactive immune system will immediately notice a sudden change in the body's response, which we generally call allergic symptoms. Some may notice them after 2 to 3 days. Ideally, you should wait for a couple of days to see if any food is acting like a trigger. So go slowly and start with one food item at a time.

It's best to eat the trigger food item **early in the day**, the earlier the better to assess your body's abnormal response, if any. If you don't observe any changes, you can go ahead and add that food back into your regular diet now.

However, if you *do* notice a change, record the item and your body's response to it in your journal -- and then you will know that it's best to remove that item from your diet from now on!

And then you simply move on to the next forbidden food.

You can create one of your own, however for your convenience, a suggested reintroduction schedule is included next!

Suggested Plan For Reintroducing the Forbidden Foods

~

Days 1, 2, 3

Reintroduce **Eggs at Breakfast** for these three days. (If you didn't eat eggs before, try cheese or milk. The allergic reactions tend to be similar.)

1) **Watch** for any changes, and;

2) **Record** in your journal <u>whether or not</u> you noticed any reactions;

3) **Wash, rinse, and repeat** for the next month, **in three-day increments** for each of the trigger food items you removed from your diet two weeks ago.

Common allergic reactions to eggs or dairy products are:

* Hives or skin inflammation

* Nausea or stomach cramps, vomiting

* Coughing, shortness of breath or respiratory problems

Possible Severe Allergic Reactions to Eggs:

* Rapid pulse

* Swollen throat

* Intense abdominal pain

* Severe drop in blood pressure

* Dizziness

* Lightheadedness

These can be symptoms of anaphylaxis, a severe allergic reaction. This can be a life threatening emergency situation if it occurs, so get to a hospital immediately!

Days 4, 5, 6:

Try **Fish for Lunch** each day (salmon, cod, tilapia, snapper, etc.) and watch for changes. Record daily in your journal what type of fish you ate and whether or not you noticed any symptoms.

Common allergic reactions to fish are:

* Hives

* Rash

* Nausea/vomiting

* Swelling of the lips, face, hands, feet

* Itching

* Difficult breathing

* Diarrhea

* Stuffy or runny nose

* Sneezing

* Headaches

* Asthma

Days 7, 8, 9:

Have **Chicken for Lunch** on these three days and record in your journal. Yes, you are now free to eat chicken again!

Then again, let's not forget that chicken can be a potent allergy trigger. But it doesn't mean it's one of yours, because of course, allergens vary from person to person.

Common allergic reactions to chicken are:

* Hives and rashes (common)

* Nasal congestion (very common)

* Watery eyes

* Ear infections

* Insomnia

* Migraine headaches (common)

* Eczema

Days 10, 11, 12:

Have a **Glass of Wine** every night if you used to drink it at all. If not, skip to your next forbidden food item. Record what happens daily in your journal.

Common allergic reactions to wine or alcohol are:

* Headaches (very common)

* Eczema

* Runny nose

* Swelling of the eyes

* Vomiting

* Excessive fatigue

* Depression (very common)

* Diarrhea

Note: If a glass of wine's one of your favorite things, you may wonder why it's such a common allergenic. It's because wine contains sulfites, which are very potent triggers of allergic reactions. Although sulfites occur naturally during wine production, manufacturers also use them as *preservatives* to increase the shelf life of the wine.

Sulfites can also be found in beer and dried fruits. Most people who have a hyperactive immune system are allergic to sulfites.

Days 13, 14, 15:

Time to add in some **Grains at Breakfast**. Have some toast on rye bread one day and a whole-wheat bagel the next, record in your journal.

Reactions to grains are usually noticeable in as little as four hours, as the gluten found in them is a commonly known allergen.

Common allergic reactions to grains are:

* Nasal congestion (most common)

* Difficulty breathing, wheezing, shortness of breath

* Coughing

* Runny nose

* Swelling of the lips, tongue or face

* Eczema, hives, or skin rash

* Anemia

* Urinary tract infection

* Constipation

* Nausea or vomiting

* Cramping, irritable bowel syndrome

* Joint and muscle pain or stiffness.

Days 16, 17, 18:

Cook breakfast or lunch with **Peanut Oil.** If you never used peanut oil, use whatever oil you normally used. Record in your journal.

Common allergic reactions to peanuts are:

* Skin rashes, hives

* Digestive problems, diarrhea

* Vomiting

* Swelling of the lips, face or tongue

* Itching or tingling in or around the mouth or throat

* Breathing problems

* Runny nose

* Abdominal pain

* Sore throat

* Tightening of the throat

* Itchy, watery eyes

Note: Bet you didn't know that boys have a higher propensity to develop peanut allergy than girls, so men are more likely to be allergic than women. Being allergic to nuts is by far one of the most common allergies in history.

Days 19, 20, 21:

Have something **Sweet with Lunch**. In this case it's better not to be too specific, so chose something with sugar that you normally ate, pre-O Diet. Watch closely for symptoms and record your observations each day in your journal.

Now, sugar isn't usually considered an allergen, as our body breaks down everything we eat into glucose (blood sugar), right? So what gives? The *levels*, that's what. Too much sugar in the blood stream can invoke the same type of allergenic response from your immune system as a common allergen.

Common allergic reactions to glucose are:

* Bad headaches

* Nasal issues such as swelling of the sinus cavity, excess mucus

* Inflammation of the airways, wheezing or shortness of breath.

* Gastrointestinal complications like cramps, diarrhea, and bloating

* Confusion or forgetfulness

* Attention Deficit Disorder (ADHD)

* Depression

* Muscle cramps

* Joint pain

Most of the symptoms of high glucose levels can go undiagnosed for years until you O Diet and gather this information. Some of the symptoms for sugar can occur up to 48 hours after you've eaten the excess sugar. So keep that in mind and be vigilant. Your body will tell you what's going on with it.

So these were the primary foods that you will reintroduce slowly in the third step of the diet. **Just continue with this 3-day pattern until you've gone through all the forbidden foods you normally ate.** And do not forget to journal whether you noted any changes or not. It's all to do with finding the culprit through the process of elimination.

And keeping record can be extremely helpful to you for the future in case you happen to be allergic to several foods, or will need to seek more in-depth treatment with a licensed dietician, nutritionist, or physician.

Once you identify that any food creates an abnormal reaction in your body, you then know you have to remove it from your diet *for good* — or at least until someone creates a cure! It's the only way you'll be safe from allergic reactions for life, and you'll be able to drop your over-the-counter or prescription medications forever.

Your liver will certainly thank you!

Conclusion

~

So that's the Oligoantigenic Diet in a nutshell... or a potato skin, more likely. If you ask any one who's tried it, they'll tell you that the O Diet is a very *powerful* diagnostic tool for discovering your body's health and the ways in which it communicates about what you put into it.

Once you're over Step #3, you'll know everything!

It may help you to know that food allergies tend to be hereditary. And in some cases they can be quite severe. If that's the case with you, in order to effectively control your allergic reactions, I strongly urge you to consider consulting with a dietitian, nutritionist or Infections Disease physician for proper care.

The O Diet is a bit challenging, but if you care about improving your quality of life, you'll plan well and follow each step in good spirits!

Let's quickly review and summarize the 3 simple steps of the Oligoantigenic Diet.

Recap of Step #1

The first step is the **removal of the forbidden foods**. You take away foods that are considered the most dangerous allergy and/or inflammation irritants. Even a very small and seemingly unimportant food ingredient can be a long-term endangerment to your health.

Your gut will need a reprieve from the daily grind, and a chance to relax and stabilize. The whole digestive system will be allowed to heal itself during the next phase, which allows any symptoms that occur during the reintroduction of high-risk foods in Step #3 to be much easier to notice. You basically prepare yourself for the upcoming process of eliminating problem foods, which is theoretically the most important stage of the O Diet.

Recap of Step #2

Step 2 is when you **eat only the safer hypoallergenic foods** for a period of at least two full weeks. These foods are considered safer choices for people with hyperactive immune systems.

These nutritional elements will return the body to its natural state of operation. So, the sustainability of Step #2 is <u>extremely important</u>. You can't actually move to Step #3 without adhering to Step #2 with absolute precision.

Recap of Step #3

Step #3 is the process of **bringing the trigger foods back** into your diet, one at a time, to discover which foods specifically don't agree with your body. The first and second steps were about the process of relaxation and recovery, the third and final step is the stage of a potentially unpleasant discovery, as it can be uncomfortable to find out you'll need to give something up that you love eating.

Nevertheless, they're all under investigation in Step #3, and I recommend taking it slow and putting your undercover hat on! It's time to find out what's been going on with your body all your life!

A Few Tips For Managing Adult Allergy Symptoms Naturally

~

- **Herbs.** They soothe the digestive system and calm inflammation

- Try **saline nasal rinses** to clear sinuses. Prepare a solution of distilled water, non-iodized salt and baking soda. Get a Neti pot. Bending forward over a sink or basin, pour the solution through one of your nostrils and let it drain out the other.

- Nasal congestion can also be relieved with **steam inhalation.** Fill a saucepan with water, bring the water to a boil, add a few drops of any essential oil and try to inhale as much of the vapor as you can. Inhale deeply for 5 – 10 minutes. You can repeat the process 3 times daily.

- **Grape seed extract** works well as a natural cure.

• Most people notice symptoms like skin inflammation as immune sensitivity. You can **drink herbal tea**. Try green tea, licorice root, or Devil's claw to reduce hives.

• While in Step #2 of the O Diet, try and **monitor your stress levels** during this time. Work or personal stress can stimulate the production of the IgE antibodies, which are known to cause allergic reactions.

• Remember, chlorine is very irritating to the eyes, respiratory tract and the skin. If you're prone to develop allergic symptoms, you shouldn't swim in chlorine-filled water for long, or without goggles.

So, these are some of the most suitable options for relieving any allergic symptomology you may be experiencing. Feel free to experiment with them while you're on the O Diet. Some may prove to work better for you than others.

However, if you don't notice any relief or improvements, even after following the diet to a T, please make an appointment to see your primary care physician. Food allergy symptoms may seem simple or relatively insignificant, but they can be deadly over time with repeated exposure to the irritants.

Cases of anaphylactic shock or rapid swelling of the airways are severe forms of the immune system's allergic response as previously described. So if you think your condition is becoming increasingly unmanageable, your doctor's office is the place to be!

More Information About Common Allergenic Symptoms

~

Do you suffer with chronic migraine headaches? Chronic migraines are often related to the body's reaction to certain types of foods. During Step #3, be on the look out for migraines when you reintroduce foods like chocolate, yogurt, canned figs, tomatoes, pork, any seafood, ice cream, meat and vegetable extracts, nuts, fatty foods, coffee or caffeine products, citrus fruits and any cured meats.

The main chemical known to be responsible for triggering migraines is called Tyramine. Tyramine can be found in cheese, chocolate and citrus foods.

Cheese is often another food that increases the risk of migraines. Cheese can increase your blood pressure, which then increases the release of the neurotransmitter, norepinephrine.

What does ADHD have to do with your diet? Scientists say that people, particularly children with ADHD should avoid having foods that contain additives and artificial colors and flavors. These elements, as we said above, can trigger the immune cells situated in your gut to an allergic response, which can also make you sick.

Your gut can influence your brain. By this we mean gut inflammation. Food hypersensitivity can be triggers for depression, and mild to radical mood swings.

Sinus troubles? Sinus complication is one of the most common allergic reactions to food. And the most associated triggers are milk, cheese and ice cream. So be sure to watch for sinus irritation when reintroducing these items in Step #3 of the O Diet.

What about skin problems? Or other issues like eczema, hair loss, hives? Blood problems like abnormal clotting? Respiratory ailments like asthma, tonsillitis, adenoid enlargement or chronic cough? Gastrointestinal problems like loss of appetite, stomach cramps, and constipation? Irritation of the mouth, lip or tongue? Arthritis?

All of these things are common allergenic symptoms. And the Oligoantigenic Anti-Inflammation Diet is the key to finding out whether or not the foods you eat are contributing, in whole or in part, to these troublesome ailments. There's actually no better way to diagnose food allergies than through the process of food elimination as outlined here in the O Diet. To your health!

About the Author

~

Veronica Bond is a Licensed and Registered Dietary Nutritionist, a Certified Life Coach and certified fitness instructor. She lives in Washington State with her husband and 2.5 children.

Join Veronica's mailing list for helpful dietary and fitness tips, and to be notified of her new releases! Just send a blank email to:

author-veronica-bond+subscribe@googlegroups.com

Watch for the confirmation email you'll need to confirm your subscription.

Resources

Alyson Davis, RD. "Oligoantigenic Diet" CAM
Commons.org. 2013.
http://www.camcommons.org/oligoantigenic-diet-as-an-
evidence-based-cam-treatment.html (March 2014)

Elizabeth Landau. *"Why are food allergies on the rise?"*
CNN.com. 2010.
http://www.cnn.com/2010/HEALTH/08/03/food.allerg
ies.er.gut/ (March 2014)